Porphyria Disease

A Beginner's 2-Week Quick Start Guide on Managing Porphyria through Diet, with Sample Recipes

mf

copyright © 2022 Jeffrey Winzant

All rights reserved No part of this book may be reproduced, or stored in a retrieval system, or transmitted in any form or by any means, electronic, mechanical, photocopying, recording, or otherwise, without express written permission of the publisher.

Disclaimer

By reading this disclaimer, you are accepting the terms of the disclaimer in full. If you disagree with this disclaimer, please do not read the guide.

All of the content within this guide is provided for informational and educational purposes only, and should not be accepted as independent medical or other professional advice. The author is not a doctor, physician, nurse, mental health provider, or registered nutritionist/dietician. Therefore, using and reading this guide does not establish any form of a physician-patient relationship.

Always consult with a physician or another qualified health provider with any issues or questions you might have regarding any sort of medical condition. Do not ever disregard any qualified professional medical advice or delay seeking that advice because of anything you have read in this guide. The information in this guide is not intended to be any sort of medical advice and should not be used in lieu of any medical advice by a licensed and qualified medical professional.

The information in this guide has been compiled from a variety of known sources. However, the author cannot attest to or guarantee the accuracy of each source and thus should not be held liable for any errors or omissions.

You acknowledge that the publisher of this guide will not be held liable for any loss or damage of any kind incurred as a result of this guide or the reliance on any information provided within this guide. You acknowledge and agree that you assume all risk and responsibility for any action you undertake in response to the information in this guide.

Using this guide does not guarantee any particular result (e.g., weight loss or a cure). By reading this guide, you acknowledge that there are no guarantees to any specific outcome or results you can expect.

All product names, diet plans, or names used in this guide are for identification purposes only and are the property of their respective owners. The use of these names does not imply endorsement. All other trademarks cited herein are the property of their respective owners.

Where applicable, this guide is not intended to be a substitute for the original work of this diet plan and is, at most, a supplement to the original work for this diet plan and never a direct substitute. This guide is a personal expression of the facts of that diet plan.

Where applicable, persons shown in the cover images are stock photography models and the publisher has obtained the rights to use the images through license agreements with third-party stock image companies.

Table of Contents

Introduction   7
What Is Porphyria?   9
    The Various Types of Porphyria   10
What Is the Cause of Porphyria?   12
What Are the Symptoms?   14
    Acute porphyrias symptoms: 14
    Cutaneous porphyria symptoms: 15
How Do You Diagnose Porphyria?   16
    The pros and cons of genetic testing for porphyrias   17
Managing Porphyria Disease Through Diet   18
    Foods to Avoid   19
    Foods to Include in Your Diet   19
Sample Recipes for Inspiration   21
    Salmon and Asparagus   22
    Seafood Stew   23
    Baked Flounder   24
    Baked Salmon   25
    Seared Salmon   27
    Roast Broccoli and Salmon   29
    Asian Zucchini Salad   31
    Asparagus and Greens Salad with Tahini and Poppy Seed Dressing   32
    Lemon Roasted Broccoli   33
    Roasted Rosemary Veggies   34
    Macrobiotic Bowl Medley   35
    Veggie Bowl   37
    Fresh Asparagus Salad   41
    Fruit and Dark Greens Salad   43
    Garden Soup   45

Garlic Broccoli Salad	47
A 2-Week Plan	**48**
How to Set Up a Diet Plan for Porphyria	49
How to manage porphyria	51
Conclusion	**52**
References and Helpful Links	**53**

Introduction

Porphyria disease is an extremely rare genetic disorder among porphyrias, which results from a deficiency or defect of certain enzymes in the body.

Less than 100 cases have been documented worldwide, and porphyria disease only affects 1 to 5 people per million.

Symptoms can include severe abdominal pain, vomiting, muscle cramps, seizures, frequent itching, extreme sensitivity to sunlight, changes to skin pigmentation, and mental disturbances such as paranoia or sharp mood swings. In some forms of porphyria disease, the symptoms are triggered by exposure to chemicals including alcohol and barbiturates.

In other types of porphyria disease symptoms only become apparent during times of stress, fever, or after childbirth.

Since porphyria diseases often do not become apparent until maturity porphyria disease is considered a late-onset disorder.

Although porphyria disease is not known to be fatal, it can result in hospitalization and even death due to acute attacks.

In this beginner's guide, you will discover...

- What porphyria is
- The causes of porphyria
- Symptoms of porphyria
- How to manage porphyria through diet
- Sample recipes

What Is Porphyria?

Porphyria disease is an extremely rare genetic disorder that can result in painful symptoms such as severe abdominal pain, vomiting, muscle cramps, seizures, frequent itching, extreme sensitivity to sunlight, changes to skin pigmentation, and mental disturbances.

The word porphyria comes from the Greek word *porphyrias* meaning "purple pigment". The term porphyria was first used by Dr. Karl Joseph Eberth in 1878 after he identified that some substances were present in urine samples of porphyria patients.

Eberth porphyria disease then went on to use the term porphyria in three case studies and published them in 1880 in a medical journal. Eberth porphyria disease also identified two forms of porphyria which were named hepatic porphyria (now called acute porphyrias) and erythropoietic porphyria (now called cutaneous porphyrias).

Since these early days, there have been numerous changes within the medical world including the identification of eight different types of porphyrias, each with its own distinctive set of symptoms. The most common form is variegate porphyria, with about 80 percent of cases being attributed to this variant.

The Various Types of Porphyria

Generally, porphyria can be divided into two types:

Acute:

- *Acute porphyria* is a by-product of porphyria that produces porphyrins that are capable of inducing porphyria attacks.
- *Hereditary coproporphyria* is sometimes known as porphyria Variegate or PCT porphyria.
- *Variegate porphyria* results from a mutation in the PPOX gene and is responsible for about 80 percent of all porphyria cases.

Cutaneous:

- *Congenital erythropoietic porphyria*, also known as *Gunther's disease*. The main symptom of this porphyria is sensitivity to sunlight which causes skin blistering within minutes of exposure. This form of porphyria was fatal in early childhood until Dr. Elisabeth Schmutzhard discovered that simply applying sunscreen helped to avoid this reaction.
- *X-linked erythropoietic porphyria*, also known as *Günther's porphyria*, affects males almost exclusively.

The main symptom of this rare form of porphyria is extreme pain within the bones.
- ***Porphyria Cutanea Tarda***, best known simply as PCT porphyria, appears in adulthood and usually presents with skin problems including blisters, itching, and pigmentation changes. Unlike other forms of porphyria, it can be treated with drugs that help control mental disturbances caused by porphyria.

In addition to these many forms of porphyria, two types of porphyria diseases have yet to be classified as they only show some symptoms associated with porphyrias.

Mixed porphyria has been linked to a substance called aminolevulinic acid that accumulates in the blood when porphyrins build up in tissues and hereditary coproporphyria, also known as ALA dehydratase porphyria. This form of porphyria has only been diagnosed in less than 10 porphyria disease cases worldwide.

What Is the Cause of Porphyria?

Porphyria involves a problem in the production of heme, a component of hemoglobin. Heme involves 8 different enzymes and a deficit in one determines the type of porphyria.

As porphyrias are genetic disorders, the porphyria gene must be passed down from both parents if a porphyria sufferer is to develop porphyria disease symptoms. In some types of porphyria such as variegate porphyria and hereditary coproporphyria, each parent has a 50 percent chance of passing on their faulty gene to any children they have.

However, in autosomal dominant porphyrias such as acute intermittent porphyria and X-linked erythropoietin porphyria, it is more likely that only one parent will pass on porphyria genes.

Porphyrias are autosomal dominant, which means porphyria disease symptoms can develop even if a sufferer only has the faulty gene from one parent. It is estimated that porphyrias are responsible for about 25 percent of all cases of such disease symptoms in children born to parents who are both porphyria gene carriers but do not themselves show any signs of porphyria disease symptoms.

Porphyria can also be caused by exposure to porphyria toxins or porphyria triggers. Some of the most common porphyrinogens that can cause this condition include:

- Heavy metals such as lead, mercury, and arsenic
- Tobacco smoke
- Exposure to sunlight. This is especially true of porphyrias caused by aminolevulinic acid synthase porphyria
- Certain prescription drugs including barbiturates, antibiotics, and high doses of oral contraceptives
- Other porphyria toxins which may trigger porphyria disease symptoms in people with porphyrias include alcohol ingestion.

What Are the Symptoms?

Porphyrias' symptoms vary depending on the type of disease. Generally, sufferers will notice signs and symptoms of porphyrias at some point throughout their lives if they inherited an autosomal dominant porphyria gene from one parent.

However, congenital hepatic porphyria may have no symptoms until adulthood or old age when the accumulation of porphyrins in vital organs can cause liver failure.

Acute porphyrias symptoms:
- Abdominal pain and cramping
- Fatigue and weakness. Most porphyria sufferers will suffer from intermittent episodes of porphyria disease symptoms followed by spontaneous, but temporary, remission. These porphyrin attacks often occur at night or in the early hours of the morning after a deep sleep.
- Most sufferers experience an itchy feeling all over their bodies just before porphyria symptoms present themselves.
- Muscle pain or numbness

- Breathing problems
- Diarrhea or constipation
- Nausea
- Mental health issues, such as anxiety, hallucinations, paranoia, confusion, and disorientation.

Acute porphyria attacks usually last for between one and three weeks although the porphyrins may start to develop porphyria disease symptoms again after a few months.

Cutaneous porphyria symptoms:

- Blisters and skin lesions
- Sunburn-like porphyria skin conditions
- Skin porphyria disease symptoms cause porphyria sufferers to feel a porphyrin itching sensation on their skin. This itching causes porphyria sufferers to scratch their skin which can become red and very fragile
- Change in urine color to red or brown
- Excessive hair growth, especially in the affected areas on the skin

How Do You Diagnose Porphyria?

There are several porphyria blood tests, urine tests, and genetic tests for porphyria. If you suspect that you or a family member has porphyria, consult your doctor who can make the appropriate porphyria diagnosis.

Porphyria diagnosis begins with a physical examination which includes looking at your skin to determine which type of porphyria your symptoms are similar to. For example, your doctor will look at your skin and urine for signs of porphyria cutanea tarda, which affects adults and is characterized by blistering and photosensitivity.

The most common method of diagnosing porphyrias is to conduct a test for elevated porphyrins in the blood or urine. However, it's important to know that no one test can diagnose porphyria disease symptoms. It usually takes several tests before a diagnosis can be made. If you have been diagnosed with porphyria, you should ask your closest relatives to get tested too because some types of porphyria are inherited from one generation to the next.

In addition, there are genetic tests that can be used to diagnose porphyrias. One example is the aminolevulinic acid synthase enzyme test which can diagnose acute intermittent porphyria, variegate porphyria, or hereditary coproporphyria since these types of porphyrias are caused by defective alleles in the AMA gene.

The pros and cons of genetic testing for porphyrias

Pros of Genetic Testing

Diagnosing a patient with porphyria disease symptoms is often difficult because there are no specific tests to diagnose the condition. Genetic tests can help to make a definite diagnosis and will allow your doctor to provide you with a more comprehensive treatment plan. Also, if you suspect that you have a porphyria disorder, get your children tested too since genetic mutations can be inherited from one generation to the next.

Cons of Genetic Testing

Once the test results come back positive, it may cause distress and anxiety if you don't know how to cope with this information or what it means to have an incurable medical condition. In addition, some patients prefer not knowing which types of porphyria they have which is a concern again with the AMA test since it's possible to get false negatives.

Managing Porphyria Disease Through Diet

Unfortunately, porphyria disease is believed to be incurable. However, because the symptoms of acute porphyria are so intolerable, many people opt for an invasive medical treatment called hematin therapy. Hematin therapy involves infusing RBCs with higher-than-normal levels of hemoglobin to reduce or stop an attack before it begins. Hematin therapy is effective but extremely costly and requires lengthy stays in the hospital.

Besides hematin therapy, porphyria is also treated with a drug called Cholestyramine that helps to block the absorption of excess dietary tyrosine which can trigger acute attacks.

However, you can help manage porphyria through a better diet. Generally speaking, there isn't a particular type of diet you can follow to manage your Porphyria symptoms.

It is advisable to maintain a higher-than-average carbohydrate diet if you have the disease. Some foods should be avoided completely because they trigger symptoms.

Foods to Avoid

Your dietician can help list out the foods to avoid that would trigger your porphyria symptoms.

- Alcoholic beverages such as red wine and beer should be eliminated from the diet of a person with porphyria
- Caffeine-containing products like soda, coffee, and chocolate should also be avoided. Also, cut out nicotine and alcohol to reduce skin damage and support liver function.
- Foods that contain added sugar, saturated fats, sodium, and transportation fat, should be very limited or avoided.
- Avoid heavily processed foods

Foods to Include in Your Diet

After looking at the foods to avoid, you might probably be thinking of what foods to include in your diet. Aside from the listed foods below, your dietician can also recommend some suitable foods that are safe for your condition.

Foods that porphyria patients can eat include:
- Green leafy vegetables e.g. broccoli, cabbage
- Whole grains like brown rice, wild rice, oats, etc.
- Low-fat dairy products.
- Take small amounts of dried fruits
- Lots of water to stay hydrated

- Bread
- Porridge
- Nuts and seeds
- Ginger herbs
- Basil leaves

Generally, your entire diet should contain readily digestible foods that are centered around carbohydrates, nuts, and seeds.

Sample Recipes for Inspiration

Salmon and Asparagus

Ingredients:

- 2 salmon filets
- 14-oz. young potatoes
- 8 asparagus spears, trimmed and halved
- 2 handfuls cherry tomatoes
- 1 handful basil leaves
- 2 tbsp. extra-virgin olive oil
- 1 tbsp. balsamic vinegar

Instructions:

1. Heat oven to 428°F.
2. Arrange potatoes into a baking dish.
3. Drizzle potatoes with extra-virgin olive oil.
4. Roast potatoes until they have turned golden brown.
5. Place asparagus into the baking dish together with the potatoes.
6. Roast in the oven for 15 minutes.
7. Arrange cherry tomatoes and salmon among the vegetables.
8. Drizzle with balsamic vinegar and the remaining olive oil.
9. Roast until the salmon is cooked.
10. Throw in basil leaves before transferring everything to a serving dish.
11. Serve while hot.

Seafood Stew

Ingredients:

- 2 tsp. extra-virgin olive oil
- 1 cut bulb fennel
- 2 stalks celery, chopped
- 2 cups white wine
- 1 tbsp. chopped thyme
- 1 cup chopped shallots
- 6 oz. shrimp
- 6 oz. of sea scallops
- 1/4 tsp. salt
- 1 cup chopped parsley
- 6 oz. Arctic char
- 2-1/2 cups of water

Instructions:

1. Heat a frying pan on the lowest setting. Add a small amount of oil.
2. Cook the celery, shallots, and fennel for approximately 6 minutes.
3. Pour the wine, water, and thyme into the frying pan.
4. Wait for 10 minutes and allow it to cook.
5. Once much of the water has evaporated, add in the remaining ingredients, and wait for 2 minutes before removing it from the stove.
6. Serve and enjoy immediately.

Baked Flounder

Ingredients:

- 1 lb. flounder, filleted
- 1/4 tsp. salt
- 1 cup halved red grapes
- 1 tbsp. extra-virgin olive oil
- 2 tbsp. parsley, chopped finely
- 1 tbsp. lemon juice
- 1 cup almonds, chopped and toasted
- freshly ground black pepper, to taste

Instructions:

1. Preheat the oven to 375°F.
2. Place fish on a sheet tray. Season with olive oil, salt, and pepper.
3. Combine the almonds, grapes, lemon juice, parsley, 1-1/2 tsp. of olive oil, 1/8 tsp of salt, and black pepper in a bowl.
4. Bake the fish for about 3 minutes.
5. Flip the fish and return it to the oven.
6. Bake for another 3 minutes, or until the fish is starting to flake, while the center is still translucent. Don't overcook.
7. Serve immediately, topped with the grape mixture.

Baked Salmon

Ingredients:

- 2 salmon fillets
- 6 cups of fresh spinach
- 2 tsp. coconut oil
- 1/4 tsp. garlic powder
- 1/4 tsp. turmeric
- 3 large cloves of garlic
- lemon juice
- salt
- pepper

Instructions:

1. Preheat the oven to 400°F.
2. Line a baking dish with parchment paper.
3. Marinate salmon fillets in lemon juice, coconut oil, garlic powder, turmeric, salt, and pepper.
4. Let it sit for a few minutes. This may also be done the night before to help the juices and flavor get into the salmon.
5. Once the oven is ready, bake the salmon for 15 minutes.
6. Cook some of the garlic in a pan with coconut oil.

7. Add spinach and cook until ready. Season with salt and pepper to taste.
8. Take salmon out of the oven and put spinach beside it.
9. Serve and enjoy.

Seared Salmon

Ingredients:

- 1-1/2 tbsp. canola oil
- 4 pcs. salmon filets, each filet about 1-inch thick
- 1 tsp. kosher salt
- 1 tsp. ground black pepper, 1 teaspoon
- 2/3 cups shallots, thinly sliced, 2/3 cup
- 3 cups cherry tomatoes, 3 cups
- 2 tbsp. balsamic vinegar
- 1/2 cup basil leaves, torn

Instructions:

1. Preheat the oven to 500°F.
2. Use foil when lining a rimmed baking sheet, then set aside.
3. Put a tablespoon of canola oil in a large heavy-bottomed pan placed over high heat.
4. Sprinkle evenly half of the pepper and salt over the fish filets.
5. Cook the filets in the pan for 4 minutes until the sides are golden brown.
6. Transfer the filets, with seared sides up, onto the prepared baking sheet.
7. Put it in the oven and cook the filet for about 4 minutes or until you get the degree of doneness that you prefer.

8. Return the skillet to the stove, and add the remaining canola oil.
9. Add the shallots and sauté for a couple of minutes. Season with the remaining salt and pepper.
10. Add the cherry tomatoes and 1/3 cup basil. Cook until the tomatoes are soft, for about 2 minutes.
11. Add the balsamic vinegar. Stir and cook for about a minute.
12. Transfer the filets to a serving dish and top them with the balsamic vinegar-tomato mixture. Garnish with the remaining basil.
13. Serve and enjoy while hot.

Roast Broccoli and Salmon

Ingredients:

- 1 bunch broccoli, cut into florets
- 4 tbsp. canola oil, divided
- salt
- pepper
- 4 pcs. salmon filets, skins removed
- 1 pc. jalapeño or red Fresno chile, seeds removed, sliced into thin rings
- 2 tbsp. rice vinegar, unseasoned
- 2 tbsp. capers, drained

Instructions:

1. Preheat the oven to 400° F.
2. On a large, rimmed baking sheet, put the broccoli florets and toss in 2 tablespoons of the canola oil. Season with salt and pepper.
3. Roast the florets in the oven for 12 or 15 minutes. Toss occasionally.
4. Remove from the oven when the florets are crisp-tender and browned.
5. Gently rub the filets with 1 tablespoon of canola oil. Season the salmon with salt and pepper.
6. Put the salmon in the middle of the baking sheet.

7. Move the florets to the sides of the baking sheet. Roast the filet for 10 to 15 minutes or until the filets turn opaque throughout.
8. In a small bowl, combine the vinegar, chile rings, and a pinch of salt.
9. Let the mixture sit for about 10 minutes so that the chile rings become somewhat softened,
10. Add the capers and the remaining tablespoon of canola oil. Add salt and pepper to taste.
11. Drizzle chile vinaigrette over the roasted broccoli and salmon just before serving.

Asian Zucchini Salad

Ingredients:

- 1 medium zucchini, sliced thinly into spirals
- 1/3 cup rice vinegar
- 3/4 cup avocado oil
- 1 cup sunflower seeds, shells removed
- 1 lb. cabbage, shredded
- 1 tsp. stevia drops
- 1 cup almonds, sliced

Instructions:

1. Cut the zucchini spirals into smaller parts. Set aside.
2. Put almonds, sunflower seeds, and cabbage in a large bowl. Combine the ingredients well.
3. Add zucchini to the mixture.
4. In a small bowl, mix vinegar, stevia, and oil using a whisk or fork.
5. Pour the vinegar mixture all over the zucchini mixture. Toss well. Make sure everything is covered with the dressing.
6. Refrigerate for 2 hours before serving.

Asparagus and Greens Salad with Tahini and Poppy Seed Dressing

Ingredients:

- 10 to 12 asparagus stalks, washed well and sliced into ribbons
- 5 radishes, washed well and sliced thinly
- 2 to 3 rainbow carrots, peeled and sliced thinly
- 1 handful of wild spinach
- 1 small handful of microgreens, washed well
- 1 small handful of sunflower greens, washed well
- optional: a few pieces of chive blossoms

For the dressing:

- 2 tbsp. tahini
- 1 tbsp. poppy seeds
- 1 tbsp. extra-virgin olive oil
- salt
- pepper

Instructions:

1. For the dressing, whisk ingredients together in a small bowl.
2. In a separate bowl, toss salad ingredients into the mixture.
3. Drizzle dressing on salad upon serving.

Lemon Roasted Broccoli

Ingredients:

- 1-1/2 lb. broccoli florets
- 1/3 cup shredded Parmesan cheese
- 1/4 cup olive oil
- 2 tbsp. fresh basil, chopped
- 3 tsp. minced garlic
- 1/2 – 3/4 tsp. kosher salt
- 1/2 tsp. red chili flakes
- 1/2 lemon juice and zest

Instructions:

1. Preheat the oven to 425°F.
2. Line a baking sheet with parchment paper and spread the broccoli florets.
3. Season the broccoli with basil, olive oil, garlic, kosher salt, chili flakes, lemon zest, and lemon juice.
4. Sprinkle the top with parmesan cheese then put it into the oven for 20-25 minutes or until the cheese has slightly melted.
5. Serve and enjoy while warm.

Roasted Rosemary Veggies

Ingredients:

- 1/2 lb. turnips, cut into strips
- 1/2 lb. carrots, cut into strips
- 1/2 lb. parsnips, cut into strips
- 2 shallots, peeled
- 1/4 tsp. ground black pepper
- 2 tbsp. extra-virgin olive oil
- 6 cloves garlic
- 3/4 tsp. kosher salt
- 2 tbsp. fresh rosemary needles

Instructions:

1. Set the oven to 400°F.
2. Mix all ingredients in a baking dish.
3. Roast vegetables for 25 minutes until brown and tender.
4. Toss and roast again for 20-25 minutes.
5. Serve hot.

Macrobiotic Bowl Medley

Ingredients:

- 1/2 cup brown rice
- 3 cups chard, roughly chopped
- 1 cup squash, diced
- 1 cup broccoli florets
- 1 cup black beans, thoroughly rinsed and drained
- 1 oz. kombu
- 1/2 cup sauerkraut, chopped

Sauce:

- 2 tbsp. sesame tahini
- 2 tbsp. sodium tamari
- 1 clove garlic
- 1 tbsp. ginger
- 1 lime, juiced

Instructions:

1. Boil 1 cup of water.
2. Add rice and allow it to boil. Cover and reduce heat and simmer for 40 minutes.
3. Remove from heat and allow to sit covered for another 10 minutes, then fluff with a fork.
4. Place beans in a pot with kombu. Cover with water, and bring to a boil.

5. Reduce heat and simmer for 15-20 minutes. Drain and rinse after.
6. Place a steamer basket in a pot with water and bring it to a boil.
7. Add broccoli, cover, and steam for 4-5 minutes then remove, keeping water in the pot.
8. Add squash, cover, and steam for 4-5 minutes then remove, keeping water in the pot.
9. Add chard, cover, and steam for 3-4 minutes, then remove.
10. Mix all the ingredients of the sauce.
11. Serve everything on a plate and enjoy!

Veggie Bowl

Ingredients:

Cauliflower Rice and Peas:

- florets from 1 pc. cauliflower
- 1 tsp. olive oil
- 1/2 onion, chopped finely
- 1 clove garlic, minced
- 1 tsp. dried thyme
- 15-oz. can kidney beans, drained
- 1/4 cup canned coconut milk

Veggies:

- 1 large sweet potato, peeled and chopped into coins
- 2 pcs. red peppers, chopped into chunks
- 1 green plantain, chopped into coins
- 1 onion, chopped roughly into wedges
- 2 pcs. zucchinis, chopped
- 1 tbsp. olive oil
- 1/2 tsp. dried thyme
- 1/2 tsp. ground allspice
- salt
- pepper
- optional: vegetable seasoning

Mango Habanero Vinaigrette:

- 1 mango, peeled and chopped roughly

- 1 clove of garlic, chopped roughly
- 1/4 small habanero pepper, chopped roughly
- 1 tbsp. red wine vinegar
- 1 tsp. Dijon mustard
- 1 tsp. olive oil
- optional: fresh cilantro, chopped

Instructions:

To make the cauliflower rice and peas:

1. Pulse a third of the florets into a food processor. Process for about 10 seconds until the florets resemble rice kernels.
2. Transfer the cauliflower rice to a large bowl.
3. Repeat until all the florets have been pulsed.
4. Heat a teaspoon of olive oil in a sauté pan over medium heat.
5. Add the onion. Cook for about a couple of minutes.
6. Put the garlic and dried thyme. Cook for another minute.
7. Pour in the kidney beans. Stir and leave for another minute.
8. Pour in the coconut milk, followed by the cauliflower rice.
9. Cook while stirring occasionally, until the rice is slightly tender, for about 4-5 minutes. Sprinkle it with salt and pepper.

10. Once done, take off the heat and set it aside. Adjust taste if necessary.

To make the grilled veggies:

1. Toss the vegetables in a bowl or on a baking sheet.
2. Drizzle with olive oil. Add in the vegetable seasoning, allspice, thyme, salt, and pepper. Toss again to coat the vegetables.
3. If using a stove, heat a grill pan over medium-high heat. If using a barbecue grill, heat it to medium heat.
4. Cook the veggies in batches, until they are tender and have a nice char on the outside.
5. Sweet potatoes and plantains will need to cook for about 7 minutes on each side, red pepper for about 5-6 minutes on each side, and zucchini and onions for about 3-4 minutes on each side.

To make the mango habanero vinaigrette:

1. Place all the vinaigrette ingredients into a food processor, or blender.
2. Blend until the mixture reaches a smooth consistency.

To assemble the veggie bowls:

1. Place about a cup and a half of cauliflower rice and peas into a bowl.
2. Top it off with about 2 cups of mixed veggies.

3. Drizzle the veggies with 3 tbsp. of vinaigrette. Sprinkle with fresh cilantro if desired.
4. Serve immediately and enjoy.

Fresh Asparagus Salad

Ingredients:

- 1/3 cup of hazelnuts
- 4 cups arugula
- 1 tsp. ground pepper
- 4 tsp. lemon juice
- 2 tbsp. sea salt
- virgin olive oil
- 2 lbs. asparagus

Instructions:

1. Preheat the oven to 400°F.
2. Place hazelnuts on a baking tray with parchment paper. Place in the oven for 7 minutes.
3. Transfer hazelnuts to a plate. Optionally, to remove the skins, wrap the nuts in a towel and rub them vigorously.
4. Chop hazelnuts coarsely.
5. Remove the hard ends of the asparagus.
6. Place the stalks on the baking sheet you've used for the hazelnuts. Sprinkle 1 tbsp. olive oil and 1/2 tsp. of salt.
7. Bake for 8 minutes.
8. In a mixing bowl, combine pepper, salt, olive oil, and lemon juice. Mix well.

9. Place the arugula in a medium bowl. Drizzle 1/2 of the dressing over the veggies. Toss until everything is well coated.
10. Place arugula onto a platter.
11. Arrange asparagus on top. Sprinkle peeled hazelnuts on top.

Fruit and Dark Greens Salad

Ingredients:

- 1 cup watermelon
- 1 cup cucumber sliced or spiral
- 1/2 cup raspberries
- 1 sliced avocado
- 1 cup baby broccoli
- 1 cup papaya
- 1/2 cup toasted almonds
- 4 cups baby kale

Dressing:

- 1/2 cup olive oil
- 1/2 cup master tonic
- 1/4 cup goji berries
- 4 dates
- a pinch of sea salt

Tonic:

- 1/4 cup garlic, minced
- 1/4 cup onion, chopped
- 2 tbsp. horseradish, minced
- 2 knobs turmeric, chopped
- 1 jalapeno pepper, chopped
- 32 oz. organic apple cider vinegar
- 1/4 cup fresh ginger, chopped

- juice of 1 lemon

Instructions:

1. Mix all salad ingredients except almonds.
2. Toss salad.

To make the dressing:

1. Mix the master tonic, olive oil, and salt.
2. In a blender, blend goji berries and dates until smooth.
3. Upon serving the salad, drizzle the dressing on, and gently add almonds.

To make the master tonic:

1. Add all ingredients to apple cider vinegar.
2. Blend all ingredients until everything is mixed well.
3. Let the tonic sit in a jar for 1 to 2 weeks, shaking periodically.
4. Strain first before adding the leftover vinegar mixture into a jar with a cover.

Garden Soup

Ingredients:

- 1 can 14-1/2 oz. diced tomatoes in sauce
- 1 medium yellow summer squash, halved and sliced
- 1 medium zucchini, halved and sliced
- 1 lb. red potatoes, cubed
- 1 tsp. dried basil
- 1/2 tsp. paprika
- 1/2 tsp. salt
- 1/4 tsp. dill weed
- 1/4 tsp. pepper
- 1-1/2 cups vegetable broth
- 1-1/2 tsp. garlic powder
- 2 cups water
- 2 large carrots, sliced
- 2 medium onions, chopped
- 2 tbsp. olive oil

Instructions:

1. Heat oil in a large saucepan. Set heat to medium.
2. Saute carrots and onions until tender.
3. Add the potatoes and cook for another couple of minutes.
4. Follow by adding tomatoes, water, seasonings, and broth. Leave it to boil with the cover.

5. Lower the heat and uncover. Let it simmer until the carrots and potatoes are tender.
6. Once done, put the zucchini and yellow squash in. Let it cook until the vegetables are tender.
7. Serve as is.
8. You may also puree the soup in batches before serving. Pour more broth as you puree to get the consistency you want.

Garlic Broccoli Salad

Ingredients:

- 1 head broccoli, cut into florets
- 1 tsp. olive oil
- 1-1/2 tbsp. rice wine vinegar
- 1 tbsp. sesame oil
- 2 cloves garlic, minced
- 1 pinch cayenne pepper
- 3 tbsp. golden raisins

Instructions:

1. Fill water into a steamer. Bring to a boil.
2. Add broccoli. Cover. Steam until tender for about 3 minutes.
3. Rinse broccoli and set aside.
4. Heat olive oil in a skillet over medium heat.
5. Put in pine nuts. Stir fry for 1-2 minutes.
6. Remove from heat.
7. Whisk together rice vinegar, sesame oil, pepper, and garlic.
8. Transfer the broccoli, nuts, and raisins to the rice vinegar dressing.
9. Serve and enjoy.

A 2-Week Plan

Maintaining a balanced diet meal is very essential for porphyria patients. If you have porphyria disease, you should pay attention to your meal portion size. Do not overeat so you don't consume too many calories. The calories will only lead to other health problems, including obesity.

Also, always consult your dietician or health care provider when creating your diet plan. This is because nutritional needs do vary from person to person. The difference is based on lifestyle, medical history, and health conditions.

Your diet plan should consist of three square meals, daily. Creating a 2-week plan will help you organize your diet and ensure you are consuming the right foods in the right amount.

In addition to a diet plan, keep a food journal. A food journal is very important, especially if you want to lose weight regardless of the porphyria disease.

How to Set Up a Diet Plan for Porphyria

Week 1: Get rid of trigger foods

The trigger foods refer to the foods you should avoid because they trigger porphyria symptoms, making them more unbearable.

The first week should involve you getting rid of all the trigger foods. Your dietician can help you list out the foods to throw away. You can also refer to the list of "foods to avoid", mentioned in the previous chapter, as a guide.

It may be difficult to get rid of all the trigger foods at once, especially if you have gotten used to eating some of the foods. Start small to prevent them from your diet, then take them out completely from your pantry or food shelf. Also, eliminate these foods from your grocery list.

While getting rid of the trigger foods, also introduce suitable foods in your diet. So, what you are doing is getting acquainted with the appropriate foods by replacing the trigger foods.

Make a list of the right foods to include in your diet and include them on your grocery list.

At this point, you should restrict the number of times you're eating out. Except you are completely sure of the ingredients used, don't eat out. Completely avoid food or beverages that contain alcohol.

Week 2: Introduce a healthy meal plan into your diet

Now that you have gotten thrown away the trigger foods, it's time to fully focus on a healthy meal plan. You can create recipes that contain the accepted foods. Feel free to refer to the last chapter for recipes to construct your meal plan.

Buy only organic and fresh foods. Processed foods would only worsen your symptoms and make them more painful. You might be tempted to buy processed food because you are too tired to cook every day. In such a situation, it is advisable to cook your meals in large portions and preserve the leftovers in the fridge.

Nausea is a common problem for people with porphyria disease. Any food that makes you feel nauseous should be avoided.

Jot down every food intake and amount in your food diary. The food diary is very important if you want to track your progress so far. Your food diary should also contain the list of foods you have included in your diet.

Note: If you have acute porphyria and are looking to lose weight, you should consult your dietician or health provider. He/she will recommend what to eat and steps to take that will benefit you.

Since constipation is another common symptom of porphyria, make sure to drink lots of water. Water helps the digestion process to run smoothly and ensures you are always hydrated.

How to manage porphyria

Porphyria can cause very painful symptoms and make you feel uncomfortable. While it is not curable, because it is hereditary, porphyria can be managed. Treatment of porphyria varies depending on the type of disease. Managing your porphyria symptoms can help lessen the pain with very few consequences.

In addition to maintaining a healthy diet plan, you should also add exercise to it. Maintaining a healthy lifestyle can help you manage your symptoms.

Identifying, and intentionally avoiding, the risk factors can help you maintain a healthy lifestyle. These risk factors are triggers that would worsen the symptoms; they are often caused by environmental factors and increase the demand for heme production in your body. The risk factors include:

- Exposure to too much sunlight
- Physical and emotional stress
- Recreational drugs, as well as hormonal drugs
- Fasting or dieting
- Menstrual hormones
- Prolonged alcohol intake

Conclusion

Porphyria is unbearable and incurable but it doesn't mean you are condemned to die. Successfully managing Porphyria for a very long time is very possible. The best way to prevent symptoms is by avoiding triggers – including trigger foods of all forms.

Maintaining a healthy diet is one of the best ways to avoid triggers. Discuss with your dietician or health provider the best options for your condition.

We hope that this guide was helpful to you. If you found this information useful, please leave a review.

References and Helpful Links

2015-2020 Dietary Guidelines | health.gov. (n.d.). Retrieved December 4, 2022, from https://health.gov/our-work/nutrition-physical-activity/dietary-guidelines/previous-dietary-guidelines/2015.

Basic diet rules for porphyrics. (n.d.). Porphyria SA Found. Retrieved December 4, 2022, from https://www.porphyriasafoundation.org/recipes/basic-diet-rules-for-porphyrics.

CDC. (2022, June 17). Cdc nutrition. Centers for Disease Control and Prevention. https://www.cdc.gov/nutrition/index.html.

Diet and sleep advice. (n.d.). British Porphyria Association. Retrieved December 4, 2022, from http://porphyria.org.uk/diet-and-sleep/.

Diet Information for All Porphyrias. (2021). American Porphyria Foundation. https://porphyriafoundation.org/for-patients/diet-and-nutrition/diet-information-for-all-porphyrias/

DM; B. (n.d.). Treatment of acute hepatic porphyria with hematin. Journal of hepatology. Retrieved from https://pubmed.ncbi.nlm.nih.gov/3346530/

Porphyria | NIDDK. (n.d.). National Institute of Diabetes and Digestive and Kidney Diseases. Retrieved December 4, 2022, from https://www.niddk.nih.gov/health-information/liver-disease/porphyria.

U.S. Department of Health and Human Services. (n.d.). Porphyria - about the disease. Genetic and Rare Diseases Information Center. Retrieved December 4, 2022, from https://rarediseases.info.nih.gov/diseases/10353/porphyria.